COMPLETE GUIDE TO UNDERSTANDING BARIATRIC SURGERY

Mastering Metabolic, Essential Insight To Weight Loss, Recovery, Benefits, And Long-Term Health Transformation

KLEIN HOYLE

© [KLEIN HOYLE] [2024]

All rights reserved.

No part of this book may be reproduced, distributed, or transmitted in any form or by any means, including photocopying, recording, or other electronic or mechanical methods, without the publisher's prior written permission, with the exception of brief quotations in critical reviews and certain other noncommercial uses permitted by copyright law.

Disclaimer

The content in this book is based on the author's expertise and comprehension of the topic. The author has no affiliation or link with any corporation, business, or person. This book is meant to give general information and educational material only, and it should not be interpreted as professional medical advice. Always seek the advice of a skilled healthcare expert if you have any queries about medical issues or treatments. The author and publisher expressly disclaim any responsibility resulting directly or indirectly from the use or use of the information included in this book.

Table of Contents

CHAPTER 1 17
Introduction To Bariatric Surgery...................17
Definition And Purpose Of Bariatric Surgery 17
An Overview Of Obesity And Its Health Implications 18
History And Evolution Of Bariatric Surgery......19
Importance Of Consulting With Healthcare Professionals 21

CHAPTER 2 23
Types Of Bariatric Surgery 23
Gastric Bypass Surgery 23
    Procedure 23
    Benefits and Risks......................................24
    Post-operative Care...................................24
Sleeve Gastrectomy 25
    Procedure 25
    Benefits and Risks......................................26
    Post-operative Care...................................26
Adjustable Gastric Banding 27
    Procedure 27

    Benefits and Risks..................................28

    Post-operative Care................................28

Biliopancreatic Diversion With Duodenal Switch (Bpd/Ds) 29

    Procedure 29

    Benefits and Risks..................................30

    Post-operative Care................................30

CHAPTER 3 31

  Preparation For Bariatric Surgery...................31

  Pre-Operative Medical Evaluations And Tests...31

  Nutrition And Lifestyle Changes....................33

  Psychological Assessments And Counseling......34

  Setting Realistic Goals And Expectations.........36

CHAPTER 4 39

  Surgical Procedure 39

  Overview Of The Surgical Process..................39

  Anesthesia And Pain Management 40

  Duration And Steps Of Surgery 41

    1. Preparation and Anesthesia:....................41

    2. Incision and Access: 41

    3. Resection: 41

  4. Closure: 42

  5. Recovery: 42

 Risks And Potential Complications 42

  1. Infection: 43

  2. Bleeding: 43

  3. Leaks: 43

  4. Blood Clots: 43

  5. Nutritional deficits: 43

CHAPTER 5 45

 Immediate Post-Surgical Care 45

 Hospital Stay And Recovery Timeline 45

  Day 1: 45

  Day 2-3: 46

  Day 4-5: 46

 Pain Management And Medication 47

  1. IV Pain Relief: 47

  2. Oral medicines: 47

  3. Non-Medication Strategies: 47

 Initial Dietary Guidelines 50

  Stage 1: 50

  Stage 2: 50

Stage 3: 50
Stage 4: 51
Stage 5: 51
CHAPTER 6 53
Long-Term Post-Operative Care 53
Follow-Up Appointments, Monitoring 53
Nutritional Supplements And Vitamins 54
Exercise And Physical Activity Recommendations
.... 56
Emotional And Psychological Support 57
CHAPTER 7 59
Dietary Guidelines Following Surgery 59
Stages Of Post-Surgical Diet 59
Liquid Stage 59
Pureed Stage 60
Soft Food Stage 61
Solid Foods Stage 61
Importance Of Portion Control 62
Hydration And Fluid Intake 63
Avoiding Certain Foods And Beverages 64
CHAPTER 8 67

Potential Complications And How To Manage Them 67
Common Complications 67
    Dumping Syndrome....................................67
    Nutrient Deficits 67
Recognizing Symptoms Of Complications 68
    Identifying Dumping Syndrome 68
    Detecting Nutrient Deficits 69
Preventive Measures And Treatment...............70
    Preventing Dumping Syndrome 70
    Preventing Nutrient Deficits.......................70
When To Seek Medical Help?.........................71
    Emergency signs 71
    Routine Follow-ups...................................72

CHAPTER 9 75
Lifestyle Changes And Weight Management 75
Implementing Healthy Eating Habits 75
    1. Smaller Portion Sizes:...........................75
    2. Balanced Nutrient Intake:......................76
    3. Chewing properly:................................76
    4. Hydration:...76

- 5. Avoiding Empty Calories: 76

Creating A Sustainable Exercise Routine 77
- 2. Include Strength Training: 77
- 3. Find Fun things: 77
- 4. Set Realistic objectives: 78
- 5. Listen to Your Body: 78

Managing Stress And Emotional Eating 78
- 2. Create Coping Mechanisms: 79
- 3. Seek Support: 79
- 4. Practice Mindful Eating: 79
- 5. Plan: 79

Maintaining Long-Term Weight Loss 80
- 2. Continuous Learning: 80
- 3. Create a Support Network: 80
- 4. Stay Active: 81
- 5. Adapt to Changes: 81

CHAPTER 10 83

Resources And Support Systems 83

Find Support Groups And Communities 83
- Importance of Support Groups 83
- How to Find a Support Group 83

2. National Organizations: 84
Participating in support groups 84
  1. Regular Attendance: 84
  2. Active Participation: 84
Working With Healthcare Providers And Specialists 85
  Organizing Your Healthcare Team 85
    1. Surgeon: 85
    2. Primary Care Physician (PCP): 85
    3. Dietician/Nutritionist: 85
    4. Psychologist/Psychiatrist: 86
    5. Physical Therapist: 86
  Developing A Collaborative Relationship 86
    1. Open Communication: 86
    2. Follow-up Appointments: 86
    3. Adhering to Recommendations: 87
    4. Advocacy: 87
Continuing Education And Staying Informed 87
  Importance of Ongoing Education 87
  Resources for Information 88
    1. Professional Associations: 88

Staying Engaged 88
   1. Set Learning Goals: 88
   2. Join Professional Networks: 89
   3. Personal Research: 89
Conclusion 90
THE END 94

ABOUT THIS BOOK

The "Complete Guide to Understanding Bariatric Surgery" is an invaluable reference for anybody contemplating or having bariatric surgery. With obesity numbers skyrocketing and related health hazards becoming more prominent, this book serves as a complete guide, giving critical information and assistance at every step of the bariatric surgery process.

Chapter 1 introduces readers to the essentials of bariatric surgery, including its definition, goal, and historical backdrop of development. Understanding the ramifications of obesity and engaging with healthcare specialists are stressed, laying the groundwork for sound decision-making.

Chapter 2 goes into the many forms of bariatric surgery, from gastric bypass to sleeve gastrectomy, offering in-depth information on each procedure's mechanics and results. This section helps readers analyze their alternatives efficiently and make educated decisions based on their requirements and circumstances.

Preparing for bariatric surgery is a multidimensional process, as discussed in Chapter 3. From pre-surgery medical exams to psychological assessments and goal planning, readers are armed with the skills they need to confidently and successfully traverse this transformational path.

Chapter 4 delves further into the surgical technique, including anesthetic and pain management, as well as the risks and probable complications. By demystifying the surgical process, readers will be able to approach their procedure with more confidence and less worry.

Immediate and long-term post-surgery care are painstakingly explained in Chapters 5 and 6, ensuring that readers have a thorough understanding of what to anticipate throughout their recovery and beyond. From hospital stays to follow-up consultations and emotional assistance, every part of the post-surgery experience is explained clearly and compassionately.

Chapter 7 contains critical information on post-surgery nutrition instructions, stressing the significance of gradual food transitions and quantity management for best results. Readers are empowered to make smart food choices and practice healthy eating habits for long-term success.

The book also teaches readers how to spot and handle any difficulties, as described in Chapter 8. Individuals may reduce risks and actively protect their health after surgery by recognizing the warning signals and preventative steps.

In Chapters 9 and 10, the emphasis moves to lifestyle modifications, weight control, and obtaining tools and support networks for long-term success. Readers are advised to take a comprehensive approach to long-term well-being, from building sustainable workout routines to seeking community assistance.

In summary, the "Complete Guide to Understanding Bariatric Surgery" is a source of education, empowerment, and support for anyone beginning on this revolutionary path to better health and quality of life.

CHAPTER 1
Introduction To Bariatric Surgery

Definition And Purpose Of Bariatric Surgery

Bariatric surgery encompasses a wide range of surgical techniques done on obese people to assist in weight reduction. The major purpose of these procedures is to change the digestive system in a manner that restricts food intake and/or inhibits nutritional absorption, resulting in considerable and long-term weight reduction. Bariatric surgery is classified into numerous forms, including gastric bypass, sleeve gastrectomy, and adjustable gastric banding, each with its own set of processes and advantages.

The goal of bariatric surgery goes beyond cosmetic weight reduction; it is a necessary intervention for those whose obesity creates serious health concerns. Obesity-related illnesses such as type 2 diabetes, hypertension, sleep apnea, and cardiovascular disease may all be helped or perhaps resolved with this operation. Patients who lose a significant amount of weight may improve their quality of life, mobility, and lifespan. Bariatric surgery is often recommended for those with a body mass index (BMI) of 40 or higher, or those with a BMI of 35 or higher who also have substantial obesity-related health issues.

An Overview Of Obesity And Its Health Implications

Obesity is a complicated, chronic condition defined by excessive bodily fat buildup, which is harmful to one's health. It is commonly assessed using the BMI, with a BMI of 30 or more qualifying as obese. Obesity rates are growing worldwide, impacting both industrialized and developing nations. Obesity is caused by a combination of genetics, sedentary lifestyles, poor eating habits, and environmental factors.

Obesity has far-reaching and complex health repercussions. Obese people are more likely to develop a variety of medical diseases, such as metabolic, cardiovascular, and musculoskeletal illnesses. Type 2 diabetes is one of the most serious health hazards connected with obesity, owing to the body's inability to adequately utilize insulin. Another prevalent illness is hypertension, sometimes known as high blood pressure, which may lead to serious problems including heart disease and stroke. Obesity is also associated with some forms of cancer, respiratory disorders such as sleep apnea, and mental health concerns such as depression and anxiety.

History And Evolution Of Bariatric Surgery

The history of bariatric surgery begins in the 1950s when the first operations were created in response to the rising understanding of obesity as a severe health concern.

Early operations, such as the jejunoileal bypass, required bypassing a considerable amount of the small intestine to minimize food absorption, but they often resulted in serious complications and nutritional deficits.

Surgical procedures have changed dramatically throughout the decades. In the 1960s and 1970s, the emergence of gastric bypass surgery, which combines stomach reduction with a tiny intestinal bypass, represented a watershed moment. This technique not only controlled food intake but also changed gut hormones, which helped to maintain weight reduction and enhance metabolic results.

The 1990s witnessed the introduction of laparoscopic surgery, a less invasive procedure that lowered recuperation periods and surgical risks. Due to its effectiveness and safety, procedures such as laparoscopic adjustable gastric banding and laparoscopic sleeve gastrectomy have grown in popularity. Recent advances in bariatric surgery have focused on improving approaches to improve patient outcomes and reduce problems, such as the creation of robotic-assisted surgery.

Importance Of Consulting With Healthcare Professionals

Consultation with healthcare specialists is an important step in bariatric surgery. This interdisciplinary approach usually includes consultations with surgeons, nutritionists, psychologists, and primary care doctors. The first examination determines if a patient is a good candidate for surgery based on their medical history, current health, and weight reduction objectives.

Surgeons give thorough information on the many kinds of bariatric surgery, including the possible advantages and hazards of each. Dietitians evaluate the patient's nutritional habits and create a pre- and post-surgery dietary plan to ensure that they satisfy their nutritional requirements and promote optimum healing. Psychologists assess the patient's mental health and surgical preparedness, treating any underlying conditions such as eating disorders or depression that may influence the surgery's outcome.

Primary care doctors coordinate treatment, manage chronic illnesses, and ensure patients are medically suitable for surgery. This complete diagnostic approach not only assists patients in making an educated choice about having bariatric surgery, but it also lays the groundwork for long-term success by educating them about the lifestyle adjustments required to sustain weight reduction and enhance overall health.

CHAPTER 2

Types Of Bariatric Surgery

Gastric Bypass Surgery

Gastric bypass surgery, also known as Roux-en-Y gastric bypass, is one of the most popular and successful types of bariatric surgery. This method includes forming a tiny stomach pouch from the original stomach and linking it directly to the small intestine. This skips a large amount of the stomach and the first part of the small intestine (the duodenum), resulting in lower calorie absorption and decreased stomach capacity.

Procedure

The procedure usually starts with the patient under general anesthesia. Using either open or laparoscopic procedures, the surgeon staples the top region of the stomach to form a tiny pouch about the size of an egg.

This pouch is subsequently attached to the jejunum (a section of the small intestine), providing a Y-shaped connection that permits food to skip the stomach and duodenum.

Benefits and Risks

One of the key advantages of gastric bypass surgery is considerable weight reduction, which may help to ease or resolve obesity-related problems including type 2 diabetes, hypertension, and sleep apnea. However, hazards include nutritional shortages as a result of limited vitamin absorption, the possibility of dumping syndrome (rapid stomach emptying), and the typical dangers associated with major surgery, such as infections or anesthetic difficulties.

Post-operative Care

Gastric bypass patients must adhere to a stringent eating plan after their surgery. Patients are first confined to a liquid diet, gradually progressing to pureed meals, and then to solid foods. Regular follow-up visits with healthcare specialists are critical for tracking dietary intake and general health. Patients must take vitamin and mineral supplements throughout their lives to avoid deficits.

Sleeve Gastrectomy

Sleeve gastrectomy, often known as gastric sleeve surgery, is another common bariatric surgery procedure. This treatment includes removing a major section of the stomach, leaving behind a sleeve-shaped stomach around the size and shape of a banana.

Procedure

During a sleeve gastrectomy, the surgeon creates tiny abdominal incisions to insert a laparoscope and other surgical equipment. The bigger, curved portion of the stomach is eliminated, revealing a tubular pouch. This smaller stomach restricts the quantity of food that can be taken and inhibits the release of the hunger hormone ghrelin, which helps to suppress appetite.

Benefits and Risks

The advantages of sleeve gastrectomy include significant weight reduction and relief in concomitant illnesses such as diabetes, high blood pressure, and cholesterol. Furthermore, this technique does not entail rerouting the intestines, which reduces the risk of several problems associated with gastric bypass. However, hazards include staple line leaking, blood clots, and long-term nutritional deficits.

Post-operative Care

Following surgery, patients follow a similar dietary pattern to those who have gastric bypass, beginning with liquids and gradually reintroducing solid meals. Lifelong dietary adjustments and vitamin supplements are required.

Regular medical check-ups assist the patient to adjust to the increased stomach size and maintain enough nourishment.

Adjustable Gastric Banding

Adjustable gastric banding, often known as lap band surgery, involves wrapping an inflatable band around the top region of the stomach to form a tiny pouch that stores food. The band may be changed to regulate the pace of food consumption.

Procedure

The procedure is generally done laparoscopically. The surgeon wraps a silicone band around the top section of the stomach, forming a tiny pouch above the band and the remainder of the stomach underneath. The band is attached to a port beneath the abdomen's skin. This port enables the surgeon to alter the band's tension by injecting or withdrawing saline.

Benefits and Risks

Adjustable gastric banding is a less invasive and reversible bariatric surgery. The changeable nature of the band allows for individual control over food intake, which may be changed without requiring further surgery. However, weight reduction is often slower than with other treatments, and the band may slide, erode, or cause infection. Patients may feel nausea and vomiting if the band is overly tight.

Post-operative Care

Following the operation, patients will follow a diet that progresses from liquids to solids. Adjustments to the band are done depending on weight reduction and food tolerance. Regular follow-up appointments are required to check the band's location and the patient's general health. Patients must commit to long-term lifestyle modifications and may need vitamin supplements.

Biliopancreatic Diversion With Duodenal Switch (Bpd/Ds)

Biliopancreatic diversion with a duodenal switch is a complicated and uncommon bariatric operation. It combines two techniques: a restrictive component (akin to sleeve gastrectomy) and a malabsorptive component (which bypasses a large amount of the small intestine).

Procedure

The operation begins with a sleeve gastrectomy, which removes a major section of the stomach, resulting in a smaller stomach pouch. The surgeon then reroutes a long section of the small intestine, creating two independent pathways: one for food and one for bile and pancreatic enzymes. These two channels connect closer to the bottom region of the small intestine, minimizing the amount of time food interacts with digestive fluids and so lowering calorie and nutrient absorption.

Benefits and Risks

BPD/DS produces the greatest weight reduction and improvement in metabolic diseases such as diabetes, often leading to remission. However, because of its intricacy, it is associated with greater risks than other bariatric operations. Potential risks include nutritional deficits, especially those involving fat-soluble vitamins (A, D, E, and K), protein deficiency, and an increased risk of surgical complications.

Post-operative Care

Patients must follow a tight and thorough food plan to guarantee proper nutrition and avoid deficits. This includes high-protein meals as well as vitamin and mineral supplements throughout life. Regular medical check-ups are required to maintain your nutritional condition and general health. Patients must also be watchful for indicators of malnutrition and collaborate closely with their healthcare team to monitor their food and supplements.

CHAPTER 3

Preparation For Bariatric Surgery

Pre-Operative Medical Evaluations And Tests

Before having bariatric surgery, a set of extensive medical assessments and testing are required to determine that you are a qualified candidate and to reduce possible hazards. These examinations usually begin with a comprehensive review of your medical history and a physical examination by both your primary care physician and the bariatric surgeon.

The following stage is usually a battery of blood tests to evaluate your general health, such as a complete blood count (CBC), liver and kidney function tests, lipid profile, and blood glucose levels. These tests aid in detecting any underlying diseases, such as anemia, liver disease, or diabetes that must be treated before surgery.

An electrocardiogram (ECG) is often conducted to detect any heart irregularities, particularly if you have a history of cardiac problems. Some individuals may additionally need a stress test or an echocardiography to get a more complete assessment of their cardiac function. A chest X-ray may also be done to confirm that your lungs are healthy and that no respiratory diseases exist.

Endoscopy is another popular examination in which a flexible tube with a camera is placed into your mouth to check your stomach and esophagus. This aids in detecting any anomalies, such as ulcers or inflammation, that may impair the procedure. Pulmonary function tests may also be performed to assess your lung capacity, particularly if you have a history of breathing issues or are a smoker.

Nutrition And Lifestyle Changes

Making major dietary and lifestyle modifications is critical in the weeks and months before bariatric surgery. These adjustments not only help your body prepare for surgery, but they also provide the groundwork for long-term success thereafter.

One of the first stages is to adhere to a pre-surgery nutrition regimen recommended by your dietician. This diet often focuses on high-protein, low-carbohydrate meals to help you lose weight before surgery, which may shrink the size of your liver and make the process safer. You should also avoid meals heavy in sugar and fat since they might cause difficulties before and after surgery.

Hydration is equally crucial. Aim to drink at least 64 ounces of water each day, but avoid drinking with meals to minimize stomach straining. Your dietician will also advise you to take vitamin and mineral supplements to address any deficiencies and ensure you are properly prepared for surgery.

You should include regular physical exercise in your daily routine. Even modest activity, such as walking or swimming, may boost cardiovascular health, expand lung capacity, and aid in weight reduction. Gradually increase your activity level as tolerated, to exercise for at least 30 minutes most days of the week.

Psychological Assessments And Counseling

Undergoing bariatric surgery is a significant life shift, and psychological preparation is an important part of the pre-surgical process. You will most likely be asked to undertake a psychiatric examination to verify that you are mentally and emotionally prepared for the changes associated with surgery.

A certified psychologist or psychiatrist will analyze your mental health history, including any previous or current depression, anxiety, or eating problems. This examination identifies any possible hurdles to success and ensures that you have the required coping skills to deal with post-surgery lifestyle adjustments.

Counseling sessions are often advised as part of the planning process. These sessions allow you to express your thoughts regarding surgery, address any anxieties or concerns, and plan techniques for coping with anticipated stresses. Topics may include creating a healthy relationship with food, dealing with stress without overeating, and establishing a support network of family and friends.

Some programs may also include group therapy sessions where you may meet individuals who are preparing for or have had bariatric surgery. Sharing experiences and advice with peers may be quite beneficial, providing extra emotional support.

Setting Realistic Goals And Expectations

Setting realistic objectives and expectations is an important step in preparing for bariatric surgery. Understanding what the operation can and cannot do can help you remain focused and prevent disappointment.

First, it's critical to understand that bariatric surgery is neither a fast fix nor a solution for obesity. It is a weight reduction tool, and long-term success is dependent on your commitment to adopting permanent lifestyle changes. Most patients should anticipate losing 50-70% of their extra body weight during the first two years, while individual outcomes may vary.

Set SMART objectives with your healthcare team, which are precise, measurable, attainable, relevant, and time-bound. These might include meeting a weight reduction goal, addressing health issues like diabetes or hypertension, or accomplishing fitness objectives like running a 5K.

It's also critical to plan for probable issues. Weight reduction may plateau over time, and you may regain some weight. Recognizing that these are regular phases of the trip will help you remain focused.

Regular follow-up sessions with your bariatric team will help you track your progress and make any required changes to your treatment plan. Celebrate minor triumphs along the road, and remember that bariatric surgery is just the start of a lifetime commitment to health and fitness.

CHAPTER 4

Surgical Procedure

Overview Of The Surgical Process

Bariatric surgery, which is aimed to help people lose weight by altering their digestive systems, normally consists of many critical processes, from pre-surgical preparation to post-operative recuperation. The surgical procedure starts with a complete examination by a multidisciplinary team that includes a bariatric surgeon, nutritionist, psychologist, and other experts as required.

Patients are subjected to a series of pre-operative tests, including blood work, imaging investigations, and potentially endoscopic exams, to determine that they are good candidates for surgery. Pre-surgical consultations also involve in-depth conversations about the many kinds of bariatric surgery available, such as gastric bypass, sleeve gastrectomy, and adjustable gastric banding, enabling patients to make educated choices in collaboration with their healthcare professionals.

Anesthesia And Pain Management

On the day of surgery, patients are admitted to the hospital and prepared for the operation. An anesthesiologist delivers general anesthesia, ensuring that the patient remains asleep and painless during the procedure. This includes inserting an intravenous (IV) line to provide drugs and fluids, as well as placing a breathing tube after the patient is sleeping to help with breathing throughout the procedure.

Pain control is an essential component of the surgical procedure, beginning with the provision of anesthetic. Post-operative pain management involves a variety of drugs, including opioids for severe pain, non-opioid pain relievers such as acetaminophen or ibuprofen, and, in rare cases, local anesthetics supplied directly to the surgical site. This multimodal technique reduces pain and promotes speedier recovery.

Duration And Steps Of Surgery

The time of bariatric surgery varies based on the treatment and the patient's condition, but it normally lasts one to three hours. Here's a step-by-step guide to a typical bariatric surgery technique, the laparoscopic sleeve gastrectomy:

1. Preparation and Anesthesia: The patient is taken into the operating room and given general anesthesia.

2. Incision and Access: The surgeon creates many minor abdominal incisions. Through these incisions, a laparoscope (a tiny tube with a camera) and surgical equipment are introduced.

3. Resection: Approximately 75-80% of the stomach is removed, leaving behind a tiny, sleeve-shaped stomach the size and shape of a banana. This greatly limits stomach capacity and helps to minimize food intake.

4. Closure: The stomach's borders are stapled or sutured together to form a new, smaller pouch. The abdominal incisions are subsequently closed with sutures or surgical staples.

5. Recovery: The patient is transported to a recovery area and supervised while they awaken from anesthesia. Pain treatment is ongoing, and the patient is advised to get moving as quickly as possible to avoid the danger of blood clots and other problems.

Risks And Potential Complications

Bariatric surgery, like any other major operation, has risks and possible problems, although they are relatively infrequent and can frequently be adequately handled when they do occur. Some of the potential dangers are:

1. **Infection:** Incisions may get infected, as well as the abdominal cavity itself. Proper surgical technique and aftercare may help reduce this risk.

2. **Bleeding:** While some bleeding is normal following surgery, excessive bleeding may be problematic. Surgeons make efforts to prevent bleeding during the surgery.

3. **Leaks:** After the stomach is shrunk and stapled, there is a possibility of leaks from the stapled locations. Surgeons check for leaks during operation, and patients are constantly examined thereafter.

4. **Blood Clots:** Blood clots may develop in the legs (deep vein thrombosis) and migrate to the lungs (pulmonary embolism). Early mobilization, compression stockings, and blood thinners may all help lower this risk.

5. **Nutritional deficits:** Because bariatric surgery affects the digestive tract, it may impair food absorption, resulting in vitamin and mineral deficits.

Lifelong supplementation and frequent monitoring are required to prevent and treat these deficits.

6. Patients may encounter symptoms such as nausea, vomiting, diarrhea, or dumping syndrome (rapid stomach emptying). Dietary changes and a gradual reintroduction of foods may help alleviate these symptoms.

Patients who recognize these risks and work together with their healthcare team may take proactive actions to reduce problems and guarantee a successful bariatric surgery.

CHAPTER 5

Immediate Post-Surgical Care

Hospital Stay And Recovery Timeline

Patients are frequently hospitalized for 2 to 5 days after bariatric surgery. The precise period varies according to the kind of surgery performed (gastric bypass, sleeve gastrectomy, etc.) and the patient's general health. Patients are transferred to a recovery room immediately after surgery, where medical professionals check vital indicators including heart rate, blood pressure, and oxygen levels.

Day 1: On the first day, patients are closely monitored. They may feel groggy as a result of the anesthetic and will usually have an intravenous (IV) line for fluids, medicines, and nourishment. It is critical to begin moving as soon as possible, typically with the assistance of nurses, to avoid blood clots and improve recuperation. Breathing exercises with a spirometer are recommended to maintain the lungs clean.

Day 2-3: Patients continue to transition to oral fluids on the second or third day, assuming no difficulties occur. The IV line is still used to provide medications. Physical activity levels improve modestly, with brief walks about the facility. This time is critical for analyzing the body's reaction to the operation and ensuring that the digestive system begins to work properly.

Day 4-5: Patients who demonstrate satisfactory progress—tolerance of fluids, controlled pain levels, and no symptoms of complications—are ready for release. Dietary advice, wound care, physical exercise suggestions, and a follow-up visit plan are all included in the discharge instructions.

Pain Management And Medication

Effective pain management is essential for patient recovery and comfort. Patients are given pain medicine via their IV line after waking up after surgery. Acetaminophen, nonsteroidal anti-inflammatory medications (NSAIDs), and opioids are all often used as pain treatments in severe situations.

Pain Management Plan:

1. **IV Pain Relief:** Initially, medicines are provided intravenously for immediate and efficient pain relief. This might include a mix of opioids and non-opioid pain medications.

2. **Oral medicines:** As patients begin to take fluids orally, they transfer to oral pain medicines. This phase ensures that patients can adequately manage discomfort at home.

3. **Non-Medication Strategies:** Encouraging patients to participate in modest physical activities, utilizing heat

packs, and teaching relaxation methods may all assist in controlling pain.

Medications Beyond Pain Relief:

• Antibiotics are used to prevent infections at surgical sites.

• Antiemetics may help manage nausea and vomiting after surgery.

• Proton Pump Inhibitors help lower stomach acid and preserve the lining, promoting healing.

Monitoring for complications

Vigilant surveillance after surgery is critical for detecting and addressing possible problems early on. Hospital personnel conducts frequent inspections for indicators of typical post-operative issues:

Bleeding: Monitoring involves inspecting bandages for excess blood and measuring hemoglobin levels. If bleeding develops, treatment options may vary from medication modifications to further surgical operations.

Infection symptoms include fever, redness, and edema around the incision site. Prophylactic antibiotics are given, and aseptic procedures are used during wound care.

Blood Clots: Deep vein thrombosis (DVT) is a danger after surgery. Patients are urged to move often, and compression devices may be used on the legs to improve circulation. Anticoagulants might be prescribed.

Leaks: Anastomotic leaks are a serious problem caused by surgical connections in the digestive system failing to heal correctly. Symptoms include severe stomach discomfort, fever, and a racing heart. If a leak is detected, diagnostic testing like CT scans is conducted, and surgery may be required.

Initial Dietary Guidelines

Dietary progression after surgery is deliberate and progressive, allowing the digestive system to repair and adjust to its new configuration.

Stage 1: Clear Liquids (Days 1-2): Patients are only allowed clear liquids for the first two days following surgery. This includes water, broth, sugar-free gelatin, and electrolyte beverages. The idea is to keep hydrated while putting a little strain on the stomach.

Stage 2: Full Liquids (Weeks 1-2): Patients go to full liquids such as protein drinks, milk, and strained soups. This stage focuses on staying hydrated and adding protein to aid with recovery.

Stage 3: Pureed Foods (Weeks 3-4): Around the third week, pureed foods like meats, vegetables, and fruits are introduced. To minimize stomach upset, the food stays smooth.

Stage 4: Soft meals (Weeks 5–6): Soft meals like scrambled eggs, soft fruits, and cooked vegetables are progressively introduced. Patients are urged to eat slowly and completely.

Stage 5: Solid meals (Week 7 onwards): By the seventh week, patients may begin to incorporate modest quantities of solid meals. The emphasis is on high-protein, low-fat, and low-sugar alternatives. Portion sizes remain limited, and patients are urged to have many small meals throughout the day.

Key Considerations:

• Patients should consume at least 64 ounces of water daily, drinking carefully and avoiding drinks with caffeine or carbonation.

• Aim for 60-80 grams of protein each day to promote tissue repair and muscle maintenance.

• Lifelong supplementation of vitamins and minerals, such as vitamin B12, iron, calcium, and vitamin D, prevents deficits caused by poor digestion and absorption.

By following these instructions, patients may aid in their recovery and lay the groundwork for long-term success in their weight reduction quest.

CHAPTER 6

Long-Term Post-Operative Care

Follow-Up Appointments, Monitoring

Follow-up consultations and monitoring are critical components of long-term bariatric surgery therapy. Following the first recovery phase, patients are often scheduled to see their bariatric surgeon, dietician, and, on occasion, a psychologist or other expert. These consultations are critical for monitoring weight reduction progress, determining nutritional health, and recognizing any issues early on.

Follow-up visits are often more frequent in the first year following surgery, occurring at one month, three months, six months, and twelve months. During these appointments, the healthcare professional will assess the patient's weight, and vital signs, and maybe do blood tests to screen for vitamin and mineral deficiencies.

After the first year, yearly check-ups are needed to guarantee long-term health and weight control.

Monitoring encompasses not just the patient's physical health but also their adherence to food restrictions, exercise regimens, and general lifestyle modifications. The healthcare team may modify the suggestions depending on the patient's progress and any new health concerns. Regular follow-ups highlight the necessity of adhering to recommended routines and allow for the early discovery of problems such as dietary deficiencies, gastrointestinal disorders, or mental health concerns.

Nutritional Supplements And Vitamins

The body's capacity to absorb nutrients may be greatly diminished after bariatric surgery, thus nutritional supplements and vitamins are an important aspect of long-term treatment.

Patients often need particular supplements to avoid deficiencies and promote overall health.

A daily multivitamin, calcium with vitamin D, vitamin B12, iron, and, on occasion, extra vitamins and minerals depending on individual requirements are all common supplements. For example, calcium citrate is often favored over calcium carbonate due to improved absorption in the changed digestive system after surgery. If oral absorption is limited, vitamin B12 may be delivered by sublingual pill or injection.

Patients must closely stick to their supplement regimen and have their nutritional levels evaluated regularly via blood testing. Supplement doses may need to be adjusted depending on the findings of these tests. To enhance absorption, supplements should be taken at various times of the day, such as calcium and iron supplements, to minimize interference with absorption.

Exercise And Physical Activity Recommendations

Exercise and physical exercise are essential for optimal long-term results after bariatric surgery. Regular physical exercise aids in weight reduction, improves cardiovascular health, increases muscular tone, and benefits mental wellness.

Post-surgery patients should begin with simple exercises like walking and progressively increase the intensity and duration of exercise as they heal. Patients may resume more organized exercise routines after receiving approval from their healthcare physician, which may include cardiovascular workouts such as swimming or cycling, strength training to develop muscle, and flexibility exercises like yoga.

It is advised that patients engage in at least 150 minutes of moderate-intensity aerobic exercise per week, as well as muscle-strengthening activities two or more days per week. Tailoring the exercise program to individual talents and interests may boost adherence and make physical activity a long-term part of everyday life. Participating in a range of activities may also assist in alleviating boredom and lower the chance of harm.

Emotional And Psychological Support

Emotional and psychological assistance are critical components of long-term care after bariatric surgery. Weight reduction surgery may cause substantial emotional changes and problems, such as body image concerns, changes in personal relationships, and the stress of adjusting to new lifestyle patterns.

Patients may benefit from continuing counseling or treatment with a psychologist who specializes in bariatric care. Support groups, whether in person or online, may create a sense of connection among people who understand the special difficulties that come after surgery.

These communities provide a forum for sharing experiences, exchanging advice, and receiving support.

Patients must address any underlying emotional or psychological disorders that may have led to their obesity. Creating appropriate coping methods for stress, anxiety, and depression is critical for long-term success. Meditation and stress-reduction strategies are examples of mindfulness activities that might be useful.

Healthcare experts may also suggest ways to boost self-esteem and body image, such as cognitive-behavioral therapy (CBT) or participating in activities that boost self-worth and confidence. Regular mental health assessments as part of follow-up treatment ensure that patients get complete care for their physical and emotional well-being.

CHAPTER 7
Dietary Guidelines Following Surgery

Stages Of Post-Surgical Diet

Bariatric surgery drastically affects the digestive system, needing a properly planned diet for appropriate recovery and adaption. This nutritional evolution is often classified into four stages: liquid, pureed, soft, and solid meals. Each step is critical for ensuring a seamless return to a normal diet while supporting the smaller stomach size and changed digestive process.

Liquid Stage

The liquid stage starts immediately after surgery and usually lasts one to two weeks. The main goal during this time is to keep the patient hydrated while allowing the stomach to recover without stress. Patients are often recommended to start with clear liquids like water, broth, and sugar-free gelatin before progressing to more nutrient-dense liquids like protein shakes, skim milk, and low-sugar juice. Sips should be taken carefully to minimize pain or pressure at the surgery site. Caffeine, carbonated beverages, and sugary drinks should be avoided since they may irritate and hinder recovery.

Pureed Stage

Following the first liquid stage, patients go to the pureed stage, which normally lasts two to four weeks. During this time, the diet consists mostly of smooth, blended meals that do not need chewing. Pureed meats, vegetables, fruits, and dairy products such as yogurt and cottage cheese are among examples. Patients should continue to ingest modest quantities, aiming for a consistency similar to baby food. Adding protein powders to pureed meals may assist in meeting protein needs. It is critical to avoid meals containing seeds, nuts, or any abrasive texture that may strain the digestive system.

Soft Food Stage

The soft foods period often starts during the fifth-week post-surgery and may last several weeks. During this period, patients may begin introducing soft, readily chewable meals into their diet. Scrambled eggs, soft fruits (like bananas and peaches), cooked vegetables, soft meats (such as fish or poultry), and tofu are also suitable alternatives. Chewing food completely is critical for digesting and avoiding obstructions. Patients should continue to eat modest, regular meals to prevent overpowering their stomachs.

Solid Foods Stage

Patients may start eating solid meals again around eight weeks following surgery. During this period, a range of solid meals is progressively introduced, to maintain good tolerance. High-protein meals should remain a top priority, with a focus on portion management and careful chewing. Patients should try new meals one at a time to see how their bodies respond and discover any intolerances or sensitivities. Tough meats, bread, fibrous vegetables, and other difficult-to-digest meals should be avoided initially since they might create pain or difficulties.

Importance Of Portion Control

Portion management is an essential part of the post-bariatric surgery diet. Overeating due to the considerably decreased stomach size might cause pain, vomiting, or even straining of the stomach pouch, undermining the surgery's efficacy. Patients are usually encouraged to consume extremely tiny quantities, frequently just a few ounces every meal, and to eat slowly so that the stomach can communicate fullness to the brain.

Using smaller plates and utensils allows you to visibly and physically regulate portion sizes. Furthermore, mindful eating activities, such as paying complete attention to the meal without interruptions, might help identify fullness signals.

Patients should learn to discriminate between hunger and other factors, such as stress or boredom, that may lead to eating.

Hydration And Fluid Intake

Hydration is another important aspect of the post-surgical diet. Because the stomach's capacity is restricted, patients must drink fluids regularly throughout the day to maintain their hydration requirements without flooding their stomachs. It is typically suggested to drink at least 64 ounces of fluid each day, with a concentration of water and other non-caloric, caffeine-free liquids.

Patients should avoid drinking big quantities at once and refrain from drinking fluids 30 minutes before or after meals to avoid straining the stomach and ensure adequate nutritional absorption. Sugar-free popsicles, herbal teas, and diluted juices may provide additional hydration alternatives. Monitoring urine color may be a useful approach to determining hydration levels;

light yellow is usually indicative of sufficient hydration.

Avoiding Certain Foods And Beverages

Patients who have had bariatric surgery must avoid particular meals and drinks to recover fully and prevent problems. High-sugar meals and beverages, such as candy, cakes, sodas, and fruit juices, may cause dumping syndrome—a disease in which food travels too fast through the stomach and intestines, resulting in symptoms such as nausea, diarrhea, and vertigo.

Dishes heavy in fat and oil, such as fried dishes, sausages, and bacon, should be avoided since they are difficult to digest and may induce gastrointestinal discomfort. Carbonated drinks are also troublesome since they may produce gas, bloating, and discomfort.

Furthermore, patients should avoid tough meats, fibrous vegetables (such as celery or asparagus), nuts, seeds, popcorn, and any other items that may cause a blockage in the digestive system. Alcohol should be avoided or taken with great care due to heightened sensitivity and altered metabolism after surgery. Each patient's tolerance varies, therefore working closely with a healthcare physician or dietician is essential for tailoring the diet accordingly.

CHAPTER 8

Potential Complications And How To Manage Them

Common Complications

Dumping Syndrome

Dumping syndrome is a frequent consequence of bariatric surgery, namely gastric bypass. It happens when food passes too fast from the stomach to the small intestine, producing symptoms such as nausea, vomiting, diarrhea, and abdominal cramps. There are two types of dumping syndromes: early and late. Early dumping occurs 10-30 minutes after eating, but late dumping occurs 1-3 hours after eating.

Nutrient Deficits

Patients are at risk for a variety of vitamin deficits after surgery due to decreased food intake and absorption. Common shortcomings include:

- Iron causes anemia, weariness, and weakness.

- Vitamin B12 deficiency may result in neurological problems and anemia.

- Low calcium and vitamin D levels may lead to osteoporosis and fractures.

- A deficit in folate, which is necessary for DNA synthesis, may lead to anemia and other health concerns.

Recognizing Symptoms Of Complications

Identifying Dumping Syndrome

Patients with dumping syndrome should be aware of the following symptoms:

- Early Dumping Syndrome causes nausea, vomiting, stomach cramps, bloating, and diarrhea quickly after eating.

- Late Dumping Syndrome: Symptoms include sweating, weakness, disorientation, and fast heartbeat 1-3 hours after a meal.

Detecting Nutrient Deficits

The symptoms of nutritional deficiencies might vary, however, some typical markers to look for are:

- Iron deficiency symptoms include fatigue, pale complexion, shortness of breath, and dizziness.

- Vitamin B12 deficiency symptoms include numbness and tingling in hands and feet, trouble walking, and memory issues.

- Symptoms of calcium and vitamin D deficiency include muscle cramps, bone discomfort, and frequent fractures.

- Folate deficiency symptoms include fatigue, mouth ulcers, and tongue swelling.

Preventive Measures And Treatment

Preventing Dumping Syndrome

To reduce the risk of dumping syndrome, patients should:

• Eating smaller, more frequent meals helps improve food digestion.

• Avoid high-sugar foods, which might worsen dumping syndrome.

• Chewing thoroughly before swallowing improves digestion and avoids fast transit into the colon.

• Limit liquid intake with meals: Drinking fluids between meals might help slow down digestion.

Preventing Nutrient Deficits

To avoid inadequacies, patients should adhere to the following guidelines:

• Adhere to Supplement Regimen: After surgery, patients are usually provided vitamins and minerals to guarantee proper consumption.

• Regular blood tests monitor vital nutrient levels, allowing for appropriate supplement modifications.

• A well-balanced diet includes a mix of nutrient-dense foods that provide a diverse range of vitamins and minerals.

• Regular visits with a nutritionist may help customize dietary regimens to specific requirements.

When To Seek Medical Help?

Emergency signs

Patients must understand when problems need rapid medical intervention.

• Persistent or severe abdominal discomfort might suggest a significant intestinal blockage.

- Uncontrollable vomiting might cause dehydration and other issues.

- Signs of severe nutrient deficiency include extreme weariness, trouble walking, severe muscular cramping, and mental disorientation, requiring immediate medical attention.

Routine Follow-ups

Regular follow-up meetings with a healthcare practitioner are required for the continuing examination and treatment of any problems. These visits usually include:

- Physical examinations are used to detect problems and assess general health.

- Provide nutritional counseling to meet dietary requirements and alter supplements as needed.

- Blood tests to check nutritional levels and identify shortages early.

Patients may successfully manage their health after bariatric surgery by remaining knowledgeable about possible consequences, identifying early symptoms, adopting preventative actions, and knowing when to seek medical attention.

CHAPTER 9

Lifestyle Changes And Weight Management

Implementing Healthy Eating Habits

Bariatric surgery is just the beginning of your road to a better lifestyle. To get the full advantages of the operation, it is essential to establish and maintain good eating habits. Your eating habits will alter dramatically after surgery due to the decreased size of your stomach. Here are some practical methods to adopt healthy eating habits:

1. Smaller Portion Sizes: After surgery, your stomach can only hold a small quantity of food at one time. This requires you to consume smaller, more frequent meals throughout the day. Eat five to six little meals instead of three big ones.

2. Balanced Nutrient Intake: Make sure your meals are well-balanced, with enough protein, healthy fat, and complex carbs. Proteins are very essential because they promote healing and help maintain muscular mass. Include lean meats, beans, dairy products, and protein supplements as needed.

3. Chewing properly: Because your stomach is small, you should chew your meal properly before swallowing. This promotes healthier digestion and avoids pain or difficulties like clogs.

4. Hydration: Drink lots of water throughout the day, but avoid drinks for 30 minutes before and after meals to avoid overfilling your stomach. Aim for at least 64 ounces of water every day.

5. Avoiding Empty Calories: Avoid foods and beverages with little nutritional value, such as sugary drinks, alcohol, and junk food. These may lead to weight regain and nutritional deficits.

Creating A Sustainable Exercise Routine

Exercise is essential for sustaining weight reduction following bariatric surgery. It not only burns calories but also improves general health and physical fitness. Here's how you can create a sustainable fitness routine:

1. Start slowly with low-impact workouts like walking, swimming, or cycling. These exercises are mild on the joints and promote endurance. Aim for 30 minutes of moderate activity most days of the week.

2. **Include Strength Training:** As you advance, include strength training routines to increase muscular growth. Muscle tissue burns more calories than fat, even while at rest. Begin with bodyweight exercises such as squats, lunges, and push-ups, then gradually add weights.

3. **Find Fun things:** Choose things that you like to make fitness a regular and fun part of your life. Enjoyment,

whether via dancing, hiking, or participating in a fitness class, can help you keep to your regimen.

4. **Set Realistic objectives:** Set attainable exercise objectives to keep yourself motivated. Keep track of your progress and celebrate tiny accomplishments to keep yourself motivated.

5. **Listen to Your Body:** Pay attention to how your body reacts to exercise. If you are experiencing pain or discomfort, adjust your actions appropriately. To create a safe and successful workout regimen, consult a fitness expert or your healthcare practitioner.

Managing Stress And Emotional Eating

Stress and emotional eating are prevalent issues that might jeopardize your weight reduction attempts. Developing methods to address these difficulties is critical to long-term success. Here's how.

1. Identify Triggers: Keep a notebook to track the circumstances, feelings, and settings that cause

emotional eating. Understanding your triggers is the first step towards controlling them.

2. Create Coping Mechanisms: Replace emotional eating with healthy coping tactics like deep breathing exercises, meditation, or participating in activities that you like. These activities may help you handle stress without relying on food.

3. Seek Support: To treat emotional eating difficulties, consider joining a support group or seeking therapy. Sharing your experiences with those who understand your situation may bring both comfort and helpful guidance.

4. Practice Mindful Eating: Pay close attention to what and how you eat. Eat carefully, relish every mouthful, and avoid distractions like television or cell phones while eating. This technique might help you identify genuine hunger and fullness signals.

5. Plan: Make nutritious meals and snacks ahead of time to prevent grabbing junk food when you're anxious or agitated. Having healthful meals easily accessible will help you make better decisions.

Maintaining Long-Term Weight Loss

Maintaining weight reduction after bariatric surgery requires continued dedication and lifestyle changes. Here are some tips to help you maintain your weight reduction.

1. Regularly monitor your weight, dietary consumption, and physical activity. This allows you to remain responsible and make the necessary changes to your routine.

2. **Continuous Learning:** Stay current on diet and fitness. Attend seminars, read publications, and interact with healthcare experts to keep your knowledge current.

3. **Create a Support Network:** Surround yourself with supportive friends, family, and experts. They may provide support, inspiration, and practical counsel as required.

4. Stay Active: Incorporate physical activity into your routine outside of scheduled training. Take the stairs, walk during breaks, and participate in energetic activities to stay moving throughout the day.

5. Adapt to Changes: Life is always changing, and your schedule may need to be adjusted over time. Be adaptable and ready to change your food and exercise routines to changing conditions while remaining focused on your health objectives.

By following these practical tips, you may get the most out of your bariatric surgery and live a healthier, more meaningful life.

CHAPTER 10

Resources And Support Systems

Find Support Groups And Communities

Importance of Support Groups

Support groups play an important part in the journey of bariatric surgery patients. They offer a secure environment in which people may discuss their stories, ask questions, and get emotional support. Being a member of a community of individuals who understand the struggles and victories that come with weight reduction surgery may boost motivation and aid in the management of post-operative lifestyle adjustments.

How to Find a Support Group

1. Hospital and clinic programs: Many hospitals and bariatric surgery clinics provide support groups to their

patients. These groups are often conducted by a healthcare practitioner and provide an organized setting for conversation and support.

2. National Organizations: Organizations like the American Society for Metabolic and Bariatric Surgery (ASMBS) often provide tools and directories for locating support groups. They may also provide virtual support sessions and webinars.

Participating in support groups

1. Regular Attendance: Consistency is essential. Regular attendance fosters ties within the group and assures continuing assistance.

2. Active Participation: Be willing to share your own experiences and listen to others. Asking questions and providing suggestions may improve the group experience for everyone.

3. Maintain a polite and discreet atmosphere. This ensures that everyone feels secure and supported.

Working With Healthcare Providers And Specialists

Organizing Your Healthcare Team

1. Surgeon: Your bariatric surgeon will be your main point of contact for surgical procedures and immediate post-operative care. They will also handle any issues that result immediately from the procedure.

2. Primary Care Physician (PCP): Your PCP will continue to look after your general health, including any non-surgical difficulties. They can help you track your progress and work with your bariatric surgeon and other experts.

3. Dietician/Nutritionist: Consulting with a dietician is necessary for developing a long-term food plan after surgery. They can assist you in comprehending your new dietary requirements, establish meal plans, and advise on vitamins and supplements.

4. **Psychologist/Psychiatrist:** Mental health specialists may assist with emotional and psychological issues connected to weight reduction and body image. They may provide treatment and solutions for dealing with change.

5. **Physical Therapist:** Following surgery, a physical therapist may assist you in developing a safe and effective exercise plan that promotes weight reduction and physical wellness.

Developing A Collaborative Relationship

1. **Open Communication:** Tell your healthcare professionals about your challenges, worries, and progress. Open communication ensures that you get the highest quality treatment.

2. **Follow-up Appointments:** Regular check-ups are essential for tracking your health and development. Make sure you attend all planned visits and complete all required exams and assessments.

3. Adhering to Recommendations: Follow the advice and directions given by your healthcare staff. This includes food restrictions, workout programs, and pharmaceutical regimes.

4. Advocacy: Do not be afraid to raise questions or seek second views if you are uncertain about any part of your treatment. Being your advocate is critical to good health management.

Continuing Education And Staying Informed

Importance of Ongoing Education

Bariatric surgery is simply one step on a lifetime path to health and fitness. Staying current on new research, methodologies, and lifestyle practices is critical for long-term success.

Resources for Information

1. Professional Associations: The ASMBS and the Obesity Action Coalition (OAC) provide essential resources such as research updates, newsletters, and conferences.

2. Subscribe to medical publications to stay up to date on the newest bariatric research. Peer-reviewed papers and articles are available in publications such as "Obesity Surgery" and "Surgery for Obesity and Related Diseases".

3. Support Groups and Seminars: Local support groups often include guest speakers and educational seminars. Attending these may give insights and practical advice for managing life after surgery.

Staying Engaged

1. Set Learning Goals: Identify particular areas in which you wish to expand your knowledge, such as diet, fitness, or mental health, and seek out resources on these subjects.

2. Join Professional Networks: If you work in healthcare, you should consider joining professional bariatric networks. These networks may provide access to special resources and networking opportunities.

3. Personal Research: Read books, watch films, and follow credible blogs and social media accounts on bariatric surgery and weight loss.

4. Periodically examine and appraise your knowledge and tactics. Stay adaptable and open to new knowledge and approaches as they become available.

By actively seeking out and participating with these tools and support networks, bariatric surgery patients may improve their chances of long-term success while also maintaining a healthy lifestyle.

Conclusion

Bariatric surgery, a revolutionary technique for extreme obesity, is a glimmer of hope for those who have struggled to lose weight via conventional methods. The end of a thorough guide to understanding bariatric surgery summarizes the diverse path that patients go through, from first consideration to long-term results, highlighting the significant effects and crucial factors involved.

Bariatric surgery is a lifestyle change rather than a procedure. The guidance emphasizes that success is dependent on a comprehensive strategy that includes pre-operative preparation, the surgical procedure, and rigorous post-operative care. To achieve and maintain weight reduction, patients must make long-term lifestyle changes, such as modifying their diets and exercising regularly. This highlights the need for a strong support system that includes healthcare doctors, dietitians, and mental health professionals.

Furthermore, the book discusses the many kinds of bariatric operations, including gastric bypass, sleeve gastrectomy, and adjustable gastric banding, each with its procedures, advantages, and dangers. This variability enables unique treatment strategies based on individual medical issues, weight reduction objectives, and lifestyle choices. Understanding these distinctions is critical for making educated decisions, and ensuring that patients' surgical choices are consistent with their long-term health goals.

Although complications and dangers are uncommon, they are an important part of the discussion around bariatric surgery. The guidance highlights the significance of educating patients about possible side effects such as dietary inadequacies, surgical problems, and the psychological consequences of fast weight reduction. Informed consent enables individuals to better manage expectations and notice symptoms that may need medical treatment, supporting a proactive attitude to health management.

The long-term effectiveness of bariatric surgery is dependent on continued medical monitoring and commitment to follow-up treatment. Regular monitoring by healthcare personnel assists in the early diagnosis of problems, ensures that dietary requirements are fulfilled, and helps patients navigate the psychological issues that may develop after surgery. The book emphasizes that bariatric surgery is not a cure for obesity, but rather a strong tool that, when paired with consistent effort and expert assistance, may result in considerable health benefits and a higher quality of life.

Finally, a thorough understanding of bariatric surgery requires viewing it as a difficult, life-changing experience. Patients and their healthcare teams must be committed, educated, and work together to achieve this. Patients are more prepared to begin on this transforming road to greater health and well-being when they have a thorough awareness of the operation, possible dangers, and necessary lifestyle modifications. This comprehensive approach guarantees that people are not only prepared to attain but also maintain their weight reduction objectives, resulting in long-term success and a healthy future.

THE END

www.ingramcontent.com/pod-product-compliance
Lightning Source LLC
Chambersburg PA
CBHW071837210526
45479CB00001B/175